End of My Journey
The Conclusion of The Children That Nobody Wanted

MARY HARRIS

Copyright © 2020 by Mary Harris
ISBN: Paperback   978-1-951670-08-5
        eBook   978-1-951670-09-2

All rights reserved. No part of this publication may be reproduced, distributed, or transmitted in any form or by any electronic or mechanical means, without the prior written permission of the publisher, except in the case of brief quotations embodied in critical reviews and certain other noncommercial uses permitted by copyright law.

Ordering Information:
For orders and inquiries, please contact:
books@authorsnote360.com
www.authorsnote360.com

Printed in the United States of America

I want to thank

Those who stood by me at

The end of my journey to the conclusion

The Children That Nobody Wanted

Years had gone by and I'm still feeling the pain of yesterday. I am trying to deal with it. My stepmom is still going strong even at 86 years old. For myself, I had experienced kidney failure. I had a fall in 2012 and broke my back while using a walker and wheelchair. The hospital wouldn't release me unless I had someone to care for me 24/7. I didn't have anyone to step up on my behalf. So, they wanted to send me to a nursing home, I felt like my past had resurfaced. My daughter had her own life with her children. She doesn't want to involve me, but I understand. Until my son came for me and moved in to help me so I can come home from the hospital. He helped me with my medication and provided me something to eat. He couldn't do personal care, so he asked his wife to move in to help me, which she did. I could never repay her for doing what she did for me. She cooked, put me in the shower; and how she did it I don't know but I am truly grateful.

Three weeks after being released from the hospital, my mom and my sister's came to help. The most beautiful thing my stepmom who I call Mrs. Edna said to me, "Do you think I would let you do this alone?" Tears flowed down my cheeks, and my heart was so full. How lucky I am to have a stepmother like Mrs. Edna, who's loving and caring.

END OF MY JOURNEY

It still makes me wonder why my biological mother couldn't love us that way. After all these years, I am still wondering why we couldn't be her first priority. Even today, no one wants to talk about it. One person told me to forget about it and go on with my life. It made ice water go through my veins by telling me to forget about it.

I called my brother crying and he said, "What's wrong sis, why are you crying?" I asked him, "Should I forget what we've been through?" His response was, "Never let anyone take away your memories about our mother walking out on us, except for God because he knows what's in your heart and mine."

It has been sixty years for me and there's not a day that goes by that I don't think about it. You must talk about it to set your mind free and have peace of mind. I love you, and I kept you all together, so our stepmom won't tell our father she couldn't deal with us. I never had a child's life. I don't regret it at all, but I wonder sometimes what it would be like for a little while. My heart is full of so much pain that I just sit and cry while wondering why she couldn't give us a little of her time. All the years had gone by and I still have no answers. Why can't I just give it up? Where are the answers? I have tried so hard to forget. I am 64 years old and now moving on. Did I forget? No, and I don't think I ever will.

My brothers are having so much anger and I just don't know how to reach out to them. We talked, and one brother told me why I should let go but I can't. With tears,

I said, "I want you to be happy even if you can't forget; because I am happy even though I haven't forgotten."

I have kids, grandkids, and great grandkids. They keep me very busy where I don't have to think about the past. Please do the same. Live in the moment. Stay away from drugs and alcohol. They can't provide any solutions for your life's tribulations. All you are doing is throwing away your life. Don't get caught up by your past. Don't let it haunt you. It will deter you to move forward.

We came a long way from being the child that nobody wanted, until this special lady came into our lives who truly loves us. Now, we are a 'somebody'. Hold your head up and never be ashamed of where you've been. I know there are so many kids that are out there who have been in the same or different situation. So many years had passed, and Mrs. Edna is still going strong. Her mind at her age comes and goes, but she never forgets to ask about all of you and how we are doing. Her words as always are. "Remember, that I love all of you."

It's 2014, I'm reaching out speaking to let others know life can change. Just look at me, a woman that had a rough life growing up and I overcame that. You can too. Sometimes, life may seem rough but just don't give up because I didn't. I had so many medical problems—from lung cancer, kidney failure, to having a broken back being an inch away from being paralyzed. I am lucky to still be here sharing my story. It's a miracle that I overcame the hurdle, but I didn't do it alone.

God was on my side every step of the way. When I fell, He lifted me up only because I know that there isn't any other God like my God. Even if I believe and trust in Him, my thought of my biological mother leaving us is still at the back of my head. I believe within my heart that God don't want me to forget. I know that God wants me to let it go, but after all these years, it still lingers. I have been trying so hard to let everything go. I cry every day when I'm alone, to the point where I'm on medication for my nerves twice a day. No one has to live this way because they can't deal with the pain for something their mother caused. Sometimes when I'm alone, all kinds of things go through my mind, so what I do is take a drink and fall myself to sleep. If only my husband were here, I would have someone to lean on to tell me that everything is going to be alright. It has been four years since he passed, and I don't have anyone in my life, maybe if I did I won't have time to think of the past.

My youngest brother has gotten so bad to the point I can't reach him. He is out there bad to the point where his family means nothing. I am so tired of trying to get him to do right. Dealing with him and my child, Betty and her girls are giving me so much trouble. It's just so much a grandmother can take. I tell my daughter every day to love her children and talk to them every day. Don't ignore them because they might be crying out for help. We listen, but we don't hear what they are saying.

END OF MY JOURNEY

Women and men take time with your children, hear what they are saying, give them hugs and kisses, and always say I love you. I talk to my grandsons to let them know to not get a mother's child pregnant and walk away—that can be very painful farther down the road. I said the same thing to my granddaughters if you have children love them and never walk away and always say you love them. I lived and experienced that when your grandmother walked out on her kids and left. It left a scar for life.

Now it's 2015, my cousin is fighting for her life. She called and wanted to see me, but I couldn't now because I was recovering from my surgery. I was afraid to travel at the time, so I promised her that I would check with my doctor to see if it was okay.

April 15, I made the trip, by then she was in the hospital. She could barely talk. I held her hand and didn't ask any questions. I told her that I love her, and that she'll be alright. I was holding back the tears 'cause I know that it's time to let go 'because now I would never hear the answers to the questions that I have been wanting for so many years. All my family on my biological mother side is gone. I have no one else to ask. My stepmom, Mrs. Edna, is the only one who's living that has answers to my questions. All she said is that she still loves you all and nothing can change that except Mary. It's time to let it go. With tears rolling down my cheeks, my response to her was, "I don't know if I can."

I share my story in workshops and speaking engagements to the youth and women and children in shelters to let them know that they're not alone. After I spoke about my life—growing up without my mother and being mistreated and dealing with so much pain, they were so thankful for me coming out to speak to them. Somewhere different from what I had been through, their testimonies were so heartbreaking and all I can say to them is, "You are not alone. There are people like you and me all over the world and we should never be ashamed of where we came from."

My oldest brother told me once why I am putting my life out there. My response to him was that I'm not ashamed of what I had been through or where I came from because we are *the children that nobody wanted* and we won't be the last. He supported me in my endeavor then and read the first book, and had a friend that read the book who can relate to my story.

On the first day of fall, I was sitting with Mrs. Edna asking her questions about my mom. All she said was, "Baby, it's time for you to let go." After all these years with no answers, and with the last person who knew gone. I looked at Mrs. Edna with tears and asked her how I can ever repay her back for all that she had done for me and my siblings. She is my hero and I love her with everything that I got. So being the mother who never made a mistake in raising us said to let it go and I will because she implored me too. And she's right it's time to let the past go. It's a life out there waiting for me, I need to go forward. It has been years since my husband died; there is no one in my life which means I must let him go also. Mrs. Edna even begged to let him go too. I still speak at the women's and children's shelters. It was still heartwarming to hear when women said how they can identify themselves in my story. Some were different from mine, and some were thanking me for coming and talking to them.

Sometimes I feel like I'm falling apart, when I'm alone my mind starts to surface. I am still living in the past of yesterday. I wonder what I am doing wrong to the point where I won't let go of the past. How can anyone, and I mean anyone who had been through what I had been through in a lifetime and still remembers the past while having so much pain. I have two brothers on my biological mother side. I'm still trying to protect them and give them good advice. Sometimes they listen and sometimes they don't. We have been *'the children that nobody wanted'* for so many years, how can any child overcome that. Today is different and I only wish I can reach every child in this world and let them see and let them know that the life that I had back in the day, and the life that I have now; I'm holding my head up and no one can say she is *the child that nobody wanted*. Each time I think about it, tears come into my eyes and all I can do is wish that the pain would go away. I can't promise that I wouldn't cry or even have pain, but I will move on with my life. I wasted so many years and time for answers that I never got. I would ask God to help me to try to find answers or let it go. And now, He said, "My child the time is now to let it go." You have come to the end of the road just keep reaching out to others and they will feel what you're feeling. This is my true-life story of my past and now it's time to let go. I still don't know how to repay my stepmother, Mrs. Edna. I thank her every day asking her is there anything she needs or wants. Her response to me was to be happy and never look back and to always remember how much she loves me.

I have a brother that was put in hospice and they called and said he had three to four days to live. Outright, I left Houston and drove to Fort Worth to be with him. I was there until he passed. He was my biological mother's son and I'm so glad I was able to be with him on his last days. By sitting on his bedside and holding his hands with tears knowing that he will be in a better place with our father, biological mom, his sisters, and all his relatives. Sometimes, we don't know the answers to all the questions, but we must let it go. I am so grateful that when we were little, and we were *'the children that nobody wanted.'* I tried my best to keep them in control, so my stepmom wouldn't say I can't deal with those kids. But being the person that she was, she never spoke a mumbling word except, "I love you as if you were my own, but I just want you all to know that you are my children and I love each and every one of you."

Before I close, I want to say to the women of the world, don't be ashamed of your body, big, medium, or small cause you are beautiful as you are. I was once ashamed of my body. I have scars that wouldn't allow me to wear certain clothes, but I realized those scars saved my life because I could've been dead somewhere in my grave. So, ladies love yourself and love your body. Don't worry about what people think because I didn't. Love all of you.

In 2016, the doctor found a spot on my lungs. I felt all alone knowing that it could be cancer. I had family and friends that could turn to, I just didn't want anyone to feel sorry for saying that poor lady like before. Until one day, I went to church and broke down without knowing, which made many people cared. I have been taking chemo. Now, I'm on medication pills which have several side effects. Weeks went by and no reaction. I thank God for giving me another chance at life. I can reach out to others who have experienced the pain that I endured. I have been lucky throughout the years from being '*the children that nobody wanted.*'

Look at me now, reach out to others to let them know they are not alone. Believe in yourself and let no one tell you differently. Life may seem rough sometimes but don't give up and you'll see what life brings. Even now, when I'm alone, I sit and wonder why a mother would walk out on her kids and never look back which caused so much pain especially when children grow up.

My journey has ended and hope someone who has experienced what I have joined my healing journey.

It's been a long journey the
children that nobody wanted

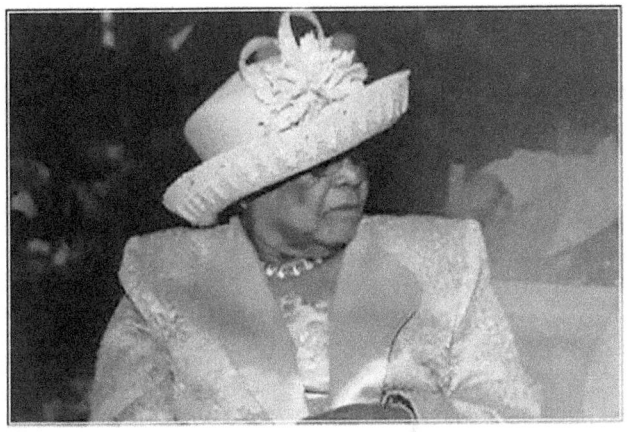

Thanks to this lady who made
me who I am today.

Love You

I was the girl nobody wanted so I fantasize what it would be like doing other things besides church and school—having a boyfriend and doing things he wanted. At the same time, we would have sex and then brag about it to his friends. So, they would make-believe they wanted me too. I was young and dumb and crazy fantasizing in a small world. Then I got pregnant and no one wanted me, I was called bad names. So, I was the girl slut who slept with any boy who wanted me in school to feel special and wanted. I couldn't believe I was letting that happen until months later I got pregnant and everyone turned their backs on me. Being pregnant in a small town brought shame to my family. I gave birth to my baby but was taken away from me. All I know is that my baby was given to a white couple who couldn't have kids of their own. My baby was multiracial because I slept with a white boy. And for a colored girl to have a baby from a white boy, that was not acceptable. I was out there on the street with nowhere to go. I can't go on living that lie. I was furious because of what my mother did—she left us. All that my father did was to find someone to help him with us, but I hurt him so bad.

I met people who introduced me to prostitution. The idea of it turned me on. It didn't take long for me to love it., I felt filled with love after all the years of emptiness I felt because no one loved me. Prostitution was my only means of surviving. I had a pimp who had me out there 24/7. My body was tired. I didn't know what to do. Then, I got pregnant again. Nine months I had the baby but I left her at a dumpster. I couldn't take her. I just wanted someone to take her and give her a good home, so she wouldn't know that her mother was a whore and a prostitute on the street in the corner day and night. Though my heart was bleeding inside, it made me not care. I was callous on what I did and on everything that was happening to me.

I kept being a whore, a good and smart one. I saved my money and opened me a whore house. I got the women off the street to come and work for me. I set them up with the richest men there were. I was a young woman with nothing to lose. I got shut down so moved into another place. If only I didn't fantasize what it would feel like doing things besides school and church. I would have not gotten pregnant. I would still have my family's love.

So, young ladies please don't fantasize of a world that you are not ready for; because it's a cold and lonely world out there. Some men would make you do things you don't want to do. When they get it, all they do is laugh and talk about you among their friends and you are left all alone.

I started on drugs and alcohol to stop the pain. I started sleeping with men doing whatever they wanted even a threesome. Whatever made me forget the hurt and pain, I'd do. Then, days later I got arrested for drugs and prostitution. I got thrown in jail for three years. I called my father yet he hanged up on me. All I wanted to do was to kill myself, which I tried with a sheet, and the person in the next cell called for help. I told her to stay out of my business, but she said, "Whatever is going on it's not worth killing yourself." I was sitting in jail thinking what would happen now when I get out of jail. I have nowhere to go except back on the street, and that was exactly what I did.

No money, hungry and cold. I had a pimp, but he didn't care. All he wanted was money. I was on the streets cold crying wishing I never wanted to fantasize what it would be like. All I did was ruin my life. I was still on the street prostituting until I met a young lady in her early 20's. I asked her what she was doing on the streets; she laughed and said, "My mother was a whore and prostitute so why can't I be?" It seems to me she knew who I was.

She called me my mother. "My blood runs in your veins I am just like you a whore prostitute and you can't stop me." I tried to explain to her why I did what I did, crying out to my daughter, "I wanted you to have a better life than I did." Yet she said, "But after all, I turned out to be just like you. The only difference about me and you is that I didn't get pregnant and put my baby in a dumpster." I pleaded, "I love you more than life itself. I wish I could change what I've done. And I ask God to forgive me for all my sins. I lost my father because I wanted to fantasize about what it would be like besides school and church."

It hurts to see my daughter turned out to be just like me. Now, I am all alone. If I had to it all over again, I would change my life and not want to fantasize.

Readers listen to your parents even though sometimes they may say things that you may not agree on. Please! Please! Please! There is a cold world out there. Trust me I have been there, and you don't want to go there.

My journey has ended
Have a bless one

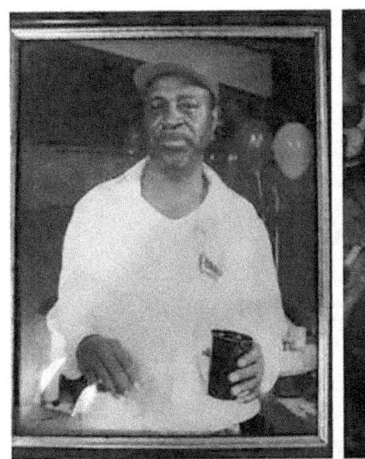
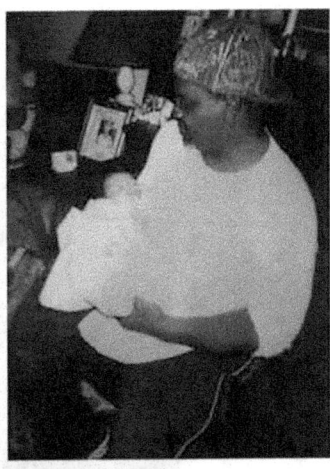
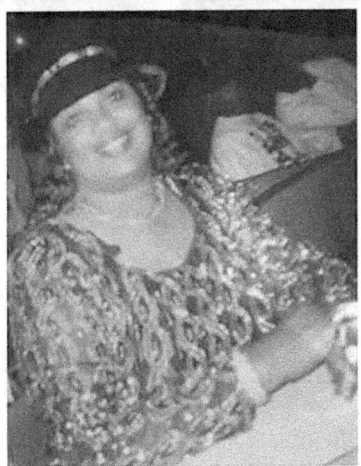

They are my last three siblings of six
from my biological mother.

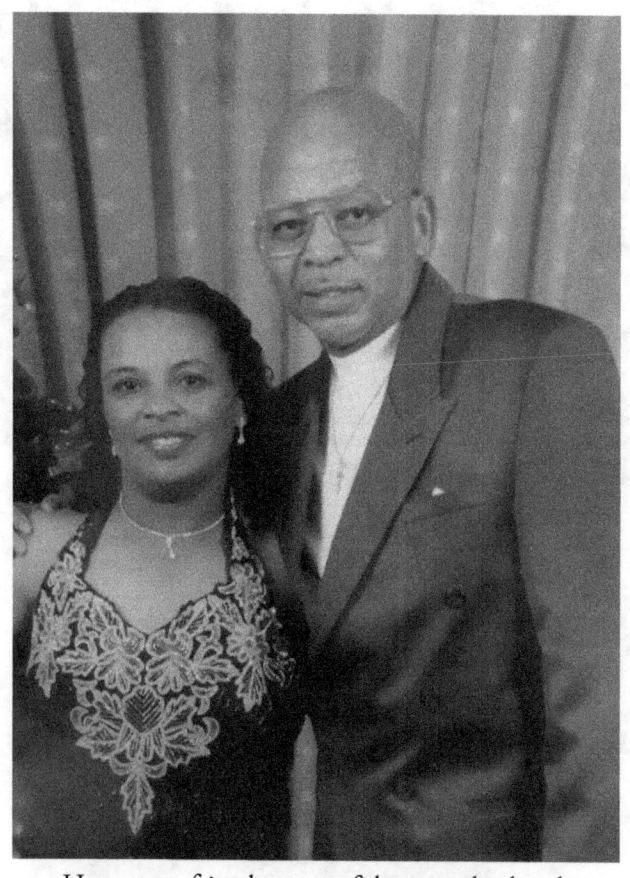

He was my friend, my confidant, my husband. He's been gone for ten years and I'm all alone. But for a moment I had forgotten that I wasn't alone cause God is with me.

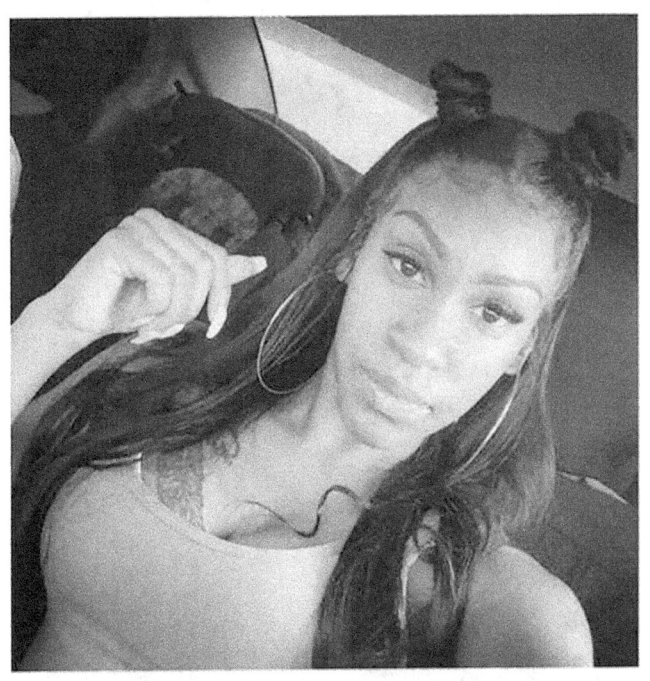

To my granddaughter I'm sending you a special thanks to helping me on this journey. I love you always, your grandmother

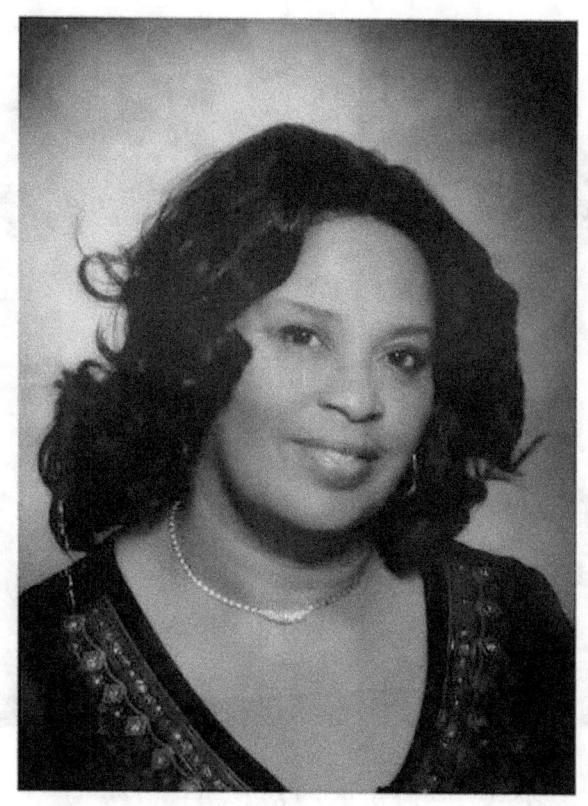

Me

www.ingramcontent.com/pod-product-compliance
Lightning Source LLC
Chambersburg PA
CBHW052129110526
44592CB00013B/1809